YOGA
A Christian analysis

John Allan

Inter-Varsity Press

Inter-Varsity Press
38 De Montfort Street, Leicester LE1 7GP, England

Unless otherwise stated, quotations from the Bible are from the
Revised Standard Version of the Bible, copyrighted 1946, 1952, © 1971,
1973 by the Division of Christian Education of the National Council of
the Churches of Christ in the USA, and used by permission.

First published 1983

British Library Cataloguing in Publication Data

Allan, John, *1950–*
   Yoga: a Christian analysis.
   1. Christianity and yoga
   I. Title
   261.5   BR128.Y/

ISBN 0-85110-443-6

Phototypesetting by Nuprint Services Ltd, Harpenden, Herts
Printed and bound in Great Britain by Collins, Glasgow

*Inter-Varsity Press is the publishing division of the Universities and
Colleges Christian Fellowship (formerly the Inter-Varsity Fellowship), a
student movement linking Christian Unions in universities and colleges
throughout the British Isles, and a member movement of the International
Fellowship of Evangelical Students. For information about local and
national activities in Great Britain write to UCCF, 38 De Montfort Street,
Leicester LE1 7GP.*

Contents

1

The East travels West

Recently Philip Wrack's column in the *News of the World* carried a paragraph about a Midlands vicar who had prevented a yoga group from meeting in his church hall on the grounds that their beliefs and practices were un-Christian and potentially dangerous. Wrack simply reported the facts and added three terse words of comment: 'Piffle, dear Vicar.'

It is probably safe to say that most readers of the newspaper would agree with him. Since the late nineteen-fifties, when it experienced an unprecedented boom in popularity, yoga has come to be accepted by the majority of the British public as a safe, ordinary, health-giving physical practice; about as occult as jogging or weight-lifting; an acceptable Women's Institute activity, alongside flower-arranging, basket-weaving and poetry reading; and nothing whatsoever to do with religion.

This is exactly the impression which the British Wheel of Yoga, Britain's leading yoga group, wishes to foster. 'Yoga is not a religion,' proclaims its *Yoga Handbook*. 'It is older than any existing religion and its ethics are to be found in all religions... No-one need fear that Yoga will conflict with his or her religion.'[1]

But traditionally Christians have not been so sure. And just this morning I have received in the post a Christian booklet which declares bluntly:

> Yoga also stems from Hinduism. The physical exercises are NOT harmless. These alone can make a person vulnerable to demonic influence.[2]

Who is right? The question has become more and more important as the influence of yoga has spread. It is virtually impossible to estimate just how many people are involved

[1] *Yoga Handbook* (Ilford, n.d.), p. 2.
[2] 'The Occult', published by Christian Publicity Organization, Worthing.

in the practice of yoga in Britain today, both because of the multiplicity of forms of yoga available – which we shall examine later – and also because of the variety of teaching outlets for it. Apart from the two largest teaching groups, the British Wheel and the B.K.S. Iyengar group, there are independent organizations such as the Sivananda Yoga Vedanta Centres, the Albion Yoga Movement and the Independent School of Yoga and Meditation. The glossy monthy magazine *Yoga Today* is available from most of the larger newsagents in Britain, and Richard Hittleman's self-instruction books and records command a wide sale. For the ordinary man in the street, there have been local authority evening classes since 1947; for the more exotically inclined, religious cult leaders such as the Guru Maharaj Ji, Bhagwan Rajneesh and Yogi Bhajan teach forms of yoga as part of their spiritual package deal. Yoga, it would seem, is getting everywhere.

The claims of yoga

Massive claims are made for yoga's effects. Psychotherapists are using meditation and *pranayama* yogic techniques to calm highly-strung patients, and physiotherapists are using the *asanas* (physical postures) for rehabilitation. When my wife and I attended ante-natal classes at our local hospital, yoga exercises were strongly recommended as the best possible post-natal therapy. Yoga is claimed to help in the treatment of stress diseases, heart and arterial troubles, hypertension and migraine. There is even a Yoga Hospital, the Kaivalysadhama Institute, at Lonavla near Bombay, combining modern medicine with a framework of Vedantist philosophy and yogic practice.

A British doctor Ann Woolley-Hart, herself a keen advocate of yoga, has been experimenting with yoga-derived techniques upon terminal cancer patients. Although cautious about claiming too much ('As yet, the number of people involved is small. It would not be proper to talk of a cure...'), her description of her results in the *Nursing Mirror* reveals how effective she feels it has been:

...The people concerned have lived longer than

expected, or are still alive. Their live's have been, or are, happy and useful. Fear has been removed and another dimension added to their personality. It may not be science, but surely it is worth doing.[3]

If terminal cancer patients are unlikely candidates for yoga, the badly crippled are even more improbable. Yet Dr Barbara Brosnan, Resident Medical Officer at a West London home for the disabled, claims that here, too, yoga confers benefits. 'People may be enabled to help compensate for – even overcome – some specific disability; they may acquire skills of protective value to their disability... The ability to exhale and inhale in a controlled fashion... may be life-saving when chest infections strike.'[4] Dr Brosnan is a convinced member of the Yoga for Health Foundation.

Thanks to the growing interest in the health-giving potential of yoga, the Foundation has now acquired a mansion-house near Biggleswade for use as a residential yoga centre. Courses organized there offer treatment to sufferers from multiple sclerosis, rheumatoid arthritis, heart conditions and stress-related diseases. In its first year of operation, some fifteen hundred people underwent 'the Ickwell experience'.

Scientists, as well as doctors, are fascinated by some of the effects yoga can produce. It has been demonstrated by several researchers that skilled practitioners of yoga can sometimes consciously control what are normally involuntary functions of the human body; pulse rate, digestion, kidney activity. EEG measurement of brain waves has demonstrated a dramatic production of alpha waves (corresponding to a state of serenity and peaceful alertness) by yogis entering a state of meditation. Grey Walter reported in 1963 that in one experiment on a Hindu doctor the alpha rhythm became so regular and monotonous that it started to look like an artificial oscillation. And the alpha state is difficult to interrupt; tests at the All-India Institute of Medical Sciences proved that alpha could continue despite

[3] *Yoga and Life* No. 8 (1980), p. 11.   [4] *Ibid.*, pp. 13–14.

deliberate distractions such as strong light, loud noises, tuning-fork vibrations, and even immersion of the hands in ice-cold water for forty-five minutes. The most that the yoga adepts did was to blink.

Dr William Tiller, the noted American physicist, now believes that 'unique information on man's internal states and perceptions have (*sic*) been lying fallow in the East for a long time'.[5] Specifically, he has developed a theory about the functioning of non-physical energies in man, which utilizes the yoga concept of seven *chakras*, or energy centres, in the body. And he is no armchair theorist. Every day, no matter how busy he may be, he spends up to an hour in meditation.

Yoga and the West

As we shall see in the next chapter, yoga concepts were introduced to the West by a number of influential Indian teachers, and yoga teaching has never strayed very far from its Indian roots. But several of the leading figures in yoga movements today are Europeans or Americans. One of the most interesting is Shri Gurudeva Mahendranath, born in London in 1911 under a very different name, who was persuaded by Aleister Crowley the magician to visit India in 1949 to learn wisdom. He stayed until 1981, when he retired to England. In the intervening years, he had lived as a Taoist priest, a Buddhist hermit, and finally a guru attracting thousands of Indian followers.

Less colourful, but equally influential, is Roy Eugene Davis, a personable middle-aged American who wears smart suits and looks like a Christian evangelist. His Centre for Spiritual Awareness is in the 'Bible belt' of North Georgia, and his writings have an evangelical ring:

Just what are we to do with the rest of our time on earth? Have we thought about it? Are we preparing for it? Do we have definite plans for our experience in the future?[6]

[5] Nona Coxhead, *Mindpower* (Harmondsworth, 1979), p. 206.
[6] Roy Eugene Davis, 'What are you doing with your life?', *Yoga Today* 5:11, p. 14.

But appearances can be deceptive. Davis has been for thirty years a teacher of the yoga techniques of his guru, Paramahansa Yogananda.

One of the brightest stars in the Western yogic firmament began to rise when in 1961 Richard Hittleman began his 'Yoga for Health' programmes on American television. Hittleman was another unlikely yogi: born in New York City, a graduate of Columbia University, American to the backbone. Perhaps because of his refreshing ordinariness, he is now, his publishers claim, 'the world's most widely read author on the subject of Yoga...his instructional albums and tapes are utilized by more students than any Yoga material ever recorded'. His influence is now transatlantic; in Europe as in the United States, 'Richard Hittleman' has become a household name.

Joseph Dippong, on the other hand, never expected to be a yoga teacher. An immigrant to Canada from Central Europe, he ran his own manufacturing business until 1970, and was no more than a typical businessman. But in November of that year he was the victim of a practical joke at a business conference he was attending, and as a result of some unfortunate horseplay he lost consciousness. Seventeen witnesses later testified that for a while 'he exhibited all the signs of a person who was clinically dead'.[7] Then he came round...and claimed to have had a life-transforming experience.

'I had been an atheist almost all of my life,' he says, 'even though I was brought up in a reasonably well-balanced Christian family.'[8] But now, believing that he had caught a glimpse of some eternal reality, he began to search for someone who could explain what he had experienced. In 1973 he gave up his business career and founded the organization he now leads – People Searching Inside – 'to show mankind their divine purpose'. But it was not until 1975, when he travelled to India to meet a yogi known as Gopi Krishna, that Dippong found the answers he was seeking. His experience had been an encounter with the *kundalini*,

[7] 'Inward Bound', brochure issued by People Searching Inside, 1978.
[8] Joseph Dippong, 'A Glimpse Beyond', *Yoga Today* 5:11, p. 24.

Krishna explained – the vital life energy that lies coiled at the base of our spine – and the awakening of this energy meant illumination, the ultimate goal of life. Today, Dippong teaches *kundalini* yoga.

People Searching Inside is an unlikely yoga group. Deeply involved in community service, it stresses such activities as reading to the blind, delivering meals to the housebound, and visiting hospitals. Its Rainbow Singers group entertains in senior citizens' Homes. These are not activities normally associated with gurus and swamis.

All of this means that it is important for Christians to know what to think about yoga. Like it or not, it is here in abundance and shows no signs of going away. Is it – as many devotees claim – the hidden wisdom underlying all religions and systems of thought? Or is it an occult delusion, a back-door sales pitch for dubious doctrines of spiritual peril? Can some of its techniques be extracted and made theologically neutral, or is it so inextricably involved with Hindu concepts that Christians should shun it completely?

Before embarking on an answer, we must step back into the past. Where did yoga come from, and what is it about?

2

Where it all came from

'On the campus of a university', comments Richard Hittleman, 'we encounter several students who are chanting Sanskrit syllables and we are informed that they are practising Yoga; a businessman tells us that in the course of his daily business activities he is applying the principles of Yoga; an elderly lady is seated in a cross-legged position gazing at the flame of a candle and we learn that she is practising Yoga; a well-known concert artist is photographed standing on his head and we read that he practises Yoga. Are all these people really practising Yoga?'[1]

[1] R. L. Hittleman, *Yoga: The Eight Steps to Health and Peace* (London, 1980), pp. 43–44.

It is a good question. The most difficult problem, in arriving at an assessment of yoga, is to work out exactly what it is. There are many different practices, techniques and philosophies – some of them mutually contradictory – in competition for the same name. The same yoga school may teach a bewildering variety of different methods; and once we start to classify, the labels change places with alarming rapidity. Some yogis claim that *laya* yoga and *kundalini* yoga are antithetical; others celebrate them as identical. To some people, *kriya* yoga is just the preparatory step to other more serious forms; others will tell you that *kriya* is a valid form in itself. Some say that Vedanta philosophy is a separate outlook on life from yoga, and does not incorporate yoga ideals; but there have been plenty of 'Vedantist' yogis, such as Sivananda, who were happy to teach all sorts of forms of yoga.

The problem of definition

Why should the situation be so confusing? There are several reasons. One is that many of the 'pop' gurus masquerading as spiritual leaders today do not know their subject very well. Words such as 'tantric' and '*kundalini*' are bandied about with little regard for their historic roots. To their credit, serious students of yoga are extremely angry about the fast-buck merchants, and firmly dissociate themselves from them. However, there are other causes of confusion rooted in the history of genuine yoga. One is that the Indian scriptures themselves are cheerfully unconcerned about internal discrepancies. R. C. Zaehner laments: 'What is a source of endless confusion in the earliest Upanishads is their readiness to make positive and contradictory statements about almost everything.'[2]

This is an attitude of mind which can puzzle the logical Westerner. But the Indian sacred books see themselves as conveying ideas which cannot really be expressed in words anyway; any material codification is bound to distort the truth, since the material world is illusory in any case (more of this later), and so contradictions can be fruitful rather than divisive.

[2] R. C. Zaehner, *Hindu and Muslim Mysticism* (London, 1960), p. 43.

Truth is eternal, too, and so no individual can claim to have seen the truth for the first time. Thus any Indian thinker, no matter how original, will endeavour to link his teaching in to some previous school of thought. It may not fit very well; it may in fact borrow rather more from somewhere else, and totally distort the teaching of the school with which it claims association; but the linking gives the teaching its credentials.

And so there are daunting problems. Any snap analysis of yoga as a simple system of exercises, or an eight-point programme for God-realization, is a caricature. Yet, despite the complexity of the subject, there are certain things that can be said.

Origins

The word 'yoga' comes from the Sanskrit root *yuj*, which means 'to unite'. Yoga is the pursuit of union: first of all, unity of consciousness within the human being himself, as he gradually quietens his involuntary impulses and takes control of his mind; then, second, union with his true Self, which lies behind the outer personality he has fabricated for himself; and, third, union with ultimate cosmic reality (or, to give it another name, God). Yoga's aims are much more than the relief of sciatica or the development of a lithe figure; they relate to the discovery of who we really are and what the universe is really all about.

As such, yoga is one of the six great *darshanas* of Hinduism. A *darshana* is a spiritual point of view with its own distinct interpretation of the Vedas (Hindu sacred scripture), and the six were identified by the fourteenth-century writer Madhava. Of the six, yoga has made by far the greatest impact on the West, and indeed it has made itself felt in the other *darshanas* too. To trace its emergence as a system of thought, we need to look briefly at the development of Indian religion.

The basic ideas of Hinduism seem to have emerged somewhere about 6,000 years ago, in the contemplations of the Rishis. These were a group of hermit philosophers living in the forests of India, who appear to have believed that there was one God, an impersonal force, indescribable

12

without any attributes. (The word now used for this concept of God is *Brahman*.) The soul of man, called *Atman* – his true self – was at one with this impersonal God, and so to find one's true self was also to find God.

These ideas are spelt out in the *Upanishads*, a confusing body of approximately 108 metaphysical speculations, written down between 1000 BC and AD 500. Man lives not once but many times, reincarnating again and again because of *karma*. *Karma* means the consequences which our actions have in fixing our destinies; we go through life piling up *karma*, and as a result we are reborn after our death. But if we achieve enlightenment, we are finally free from *karma*, and are no longer bound to the wheel of life and death. We ascend instead to the higher planes of existence outside the reach of space and time.

Thus the point of life is to achieve a realization of our real Self, which is eternal and elusive:

I have no name, I have no life, I breathe no vital air,
No elements have moulded me, no bodily sheath is my
    lair:
I have no speech, no hands and feet, nor means of
    evolution –
Consciousness and joy am I, and Bliss in dissolution.

Neither knowable, knowledge, nor knower am I,
    formless is my form,
I dwell within the senses but they are not my home:
Ever serenely balanced, I am neither free nor bound –
Consciousness and joy am I, and Bliss is where I am
    found.[3]

This poem was written centuries after the *Upanishads*, but the view of the Self is the same. The Self is the only true reality; material things are just *maya*, illusion, and salvation comes through learning to be indifferent to the material world in order to experience the Self:

When the senses are stilled, when the mind is at rest,

[3] Sankaracharya, 'Atma Shatkam' ('Song of the Soul'), quoted in B. K. S. Iyengar, *Light on Yoga* (London, 1979), p. 53.

when the intellect wavers not – then, say the wise, is reached the highest stage. This steady control of the senses and mind has been defined as Yoga. He who attains it is free from delusion.[4]

The *Upanishads* talk about God a great deal, but Savendranath Dasgupta points out that, by and large, 'this quest is not the quest of the God of the theists. This highest reality is no individual person separate from us. . . . It is, rather, a totality of partless, simple and undifferentiated experience which is the root of all our ordinary knowledge and experience and which is at once the ultimate essence of our self and the highest principle of the universe.'[5] We are a million miles from the Bible's concept of a God who is separate and distinct from his creation, and who desires a personal relationship with mankind because he himself is personal.

In fact, it was possible to adopt the leading ideas of Upanishadic religion and yet be atheist or agnostic. Buddha (as we shall see in a later chapter) derived much of his world-view from the *Upanishads,* but 'maintained a noble silence' where God's existence was concerned. And the *Samkhya* school of philosophy did without God altogether, teaching a doctrine of evolution in which nature had once existed as a single reality, but had gradually differentiated itself into more and more forms, giving birth to the world and thus to man.

Development in the East
This *Samkhya* idea of identifiable stages in creation led to the next great step in the development of yoga. Around 300 BC (though this date may be anything up to 500 years out) a scholar named Patanjali wrote the *Yoga Sutras,* the most important document in yoga's history. There may have been more than one Patanjali, and perhaps none of them

[4] The *Kathopanishad.* This quotation demonstrates a further source of confusion: the one word 'yoga' is used both for the method and for the desired result.

[5] S. N. Dasgupta, *Hindu Mysticism* (London, 1927), p. 42.

wrote the book at all; but whatever the truth, the *Yoga Sutras* simply codify yoga practice as it stood at that time. Yoga was an attempt to reverse the process of creation as *Samkhya* saw it. If creation had meant a progression from the undivided One to an infinite variety of creatures, yoga would mean a gradual integration of the human powers until all sense of individuality melted away in the blissful realization of the One. The difference between *Samkhya* and Patanjali was that Patanjali re-introduced God; when a man reached the ultimate experience of the One, he achieved union with God, the real ground of his being.

Patanjali taught that eight disciplines were necessary in yoga:

1. *Yama* – restraint – abstention from harming others, from falsehood, theft, incontinence and greed.
2. *Niyama* – observance – purity (physical and mental), contentment, mortification, study and devotion to God.
3. *Asana* – physical posture exercises, designed to bring about such mastery of the body that one's concentration is not distracted by it.
4. *Pranayama* – breath control – in order to gain mastery of the *prana,* the vital energy by which we live, which enters the body via the breath.
5. *Pratyahara* – 'withdrawal' – gaining so much mental detachment from desire that even sense-organs pay no attention to natural stimuli.
6. *Dharana* – concentration – fixing the mind on one single point – either a *chakra* (spiritual energy centre of the body) or a divine being such as Jesus or Krishna.
7. *Dhyana* – meditation – being able to direct a steady, unbroken flow of thought towards the point on which one is concentrating.
8. *Samadhi* – 'self-collectedness' – being able to see the object of concentration as it really is, without mental distortion. *Samadhi* involves several stages and ultimately provides the direct experience of God.

15

These 'eight limbs' still form the framework for most yoga systems today, however varied. By themselves, they make up a system known as *raja yoga*, which we shall examine more deeply in chapter 4. But apart from step 3 – the *asanas* – there is not a hint of what most people today visualize when the word 'yoga' is mentioned: a system of physical posture exercises. This kind of yoga, known as *hatha*, did not emerge in its full form until the fifteenth century.

Before it did, there was another important development: Tantrism. Patanjali had mentioned briefly in the *Sutras* that development as a yogi involved the development of paranormal abilities. But he was not very interested in them, and the general attitude of Indian yogis was that interest in occult powers for their own sake was wrong. They were mere by-products, to be viewed with clinical detachment. Tantrism, however, was a movement which saw the cultivation of magic powers as a worth-while end in itself, and which, instead of ignoring bodily processes, tried to use them as means of gaining spiritual power. Sexual intercourse was a case in point; many orthodox yogis had taught that habitual sexual indulgence meant a loss of spiritual power, but the Tantrics made prolonged sexual intercourse a route to enlightenment. Tantric yoga is (not surprisingly) growing in popularity in the sex-sensitive West today, and we shall return to some modern forms of it in chapter 4.

When it did emerge, *Hatha* yoga probably owed its birth to Tantrism. The new, frank interest in the body which Tantrism had brought about, and the realization that physical processes and spiritual power were closely linked, led to the writing of the *Hatha Yoga Pradipika*, in which fifteen different *asanas* were listed. Other books followed; now there are over two hundred known classical *asanas*, although thirty-two of them form the basis for the rest.

Yoga travels West
It was the end of the eighteenth century before the complicated web of ideas of Hindu thought started to fascinate intellectuals in the West. Trade with India led to increasing familiarity with her world-view, and groups such as the 'Asiatick Society of Bengal' (founded 1784) began a series

16

of translations of Oriental texts which made the Hindu scriptures available to the West for the first time. As early as 1800, Friedrich von Schlegel was proclaiming, 'In the Orient we must look for the pinnacle of Romanticism';[6] and by 1845 H. D. Thoreau, retiring to live simply at Walden Pond, looked on himself as a yogi. Certainly these men were unusual – a cultural élite unrepresentative of the population as a whole; but nonetheless their speculations prepared the Western mind for the arrival of the gurus several years later.

Queen Victoria helped, too. She described India as 'the brightest jewel in our diadem', and repeatedly received Indian spiritual leaders for audiences. One of them, Sri Govindananda Bharati, received a total of eighteen invitations to Buckingham Palace.

Perhaps the biggest impact made by any nineteenth-century Indian was made by Swami Vivekananda, a young Vedanta monk who had studied in India at the Scottish Church College and understood the thought-patterns of the West. Vivekananda did not make many converts in the West, but began some Vedanta Societies which still exist, and earned a great deal of respect from intellectual figures such as William James and Gertrude Stein. He taught four kinds of yoga: *raja,* which we have already mentioned; and *gnana, bhakti* and *karma,* which we shall examine in the next chapter.

Vivekananda did not really see himself as a missionary; he had no high hopes of winning the world for Vedanta. If his ideas spread, he told a San Francisco audience in 1900, 'the whole of humanity will become spiritual. But is it possible? I do not know. Not within thousands of years. The old superstitions must run out.'[7] The three other leading yogi figures have all been more aggressive in their approach.

Paramahansa Yogananda came to the West in 1920 to demonstrate the basic harmony of Hinduism and Chris-

[6] Quoted by Raymond Schwab, *La Renaissance Orientale* (Paris, 1950), p. 20.
[7] Swami Vivekananda, 'Is Vedanta the Future Religion?' (text printed in Calcutta, 1970).

tianity. 'As God unites all religions,' he claimed, 'it is the realization of Him as Bliss that unites the consciousness of the prophets of all religions.'[8] His Self-Realization Fellowship offers a written course of tuition leading to initiation into *kriya* yoga. and is organized from California by a group of male and female ascetics who have taken monastic vows. Yogananda himself died in 1953, but not before completing his *Autobiography of a Yogi,* widely regarded in the West as a yoga classic.

A much more prolific author was Paramahansa Sivananda, responsible for over 200 books about many different types of yoga. One of his acolytes, Swami Vishnu Devananda, now heads up over forty Sivananda Yoga Centres around the world, teaching *hatha, raja, bhakti* and *karma* yoga. Life in a Sivananda ashram is tough; the rising-bell goes off at 5.30 in the morning, and there are four and a half hours of chanting and *asanas* to survive before the first food of the day, 'brunch' at ten o'clock. There is only one other meal, and only four hours of free time in the day. Sivananda yoga is for the determined.

The fourth of the great leaders is Paramahansa Muktananda, the most influential *kundalini* yogi in the world. His name for the yoga he teaches is *siddha* yoga ('perfect yoga'), because it involves no effort on the neophyte's part. He simply allows the guru's grace to do everything for him.

Muktananda calls his initiation process *shaktipat* – a secret method of transferring his own spiritual energy momentarily to the new disciple. ('In colloquial terms,' translates Cris Popenoe, 'he zaps them.'[9]). This means that the disciples are totally dependent upon the guru for their life and spiritual power – Muktananda junkies. Gita Mehta records watching a large gathering of devotees at a film-showing of the Swami's birthday celebrations: 'people shuddered with pleasure, and stretched out their hands,

[8] Paramahansa Yogananda, *The Science of Religion* (Los Angeles 1974), p. 52.

[9] Cris Popenoe (ed.), *Inner Development* (Harmondsworth, 1979), p 385.

straining to pull the energy off the screen and into themselves.'[10]

These four leaders are all fairly orthodox expressions of
what yoga is traditionally about. More dubious forms of
'yoga' started to emerge in the late 1960s with the first wave
of contemporary religious cults. In the aftermath of the
psychedelic craze of the mid-sixties, young people who had
turned away from drugs looked for some kind of spirituality
to replace the mind-expanding experiences that chemicals
had given them. (And it should never be forgotten that the
psychedelic period was at heart a spiritual search: 'Drugs',
proclaimed its high priest Timothy Leary, 'are the religion
of the twenty-first century.') They found it partly in the
'Jesus Revolution', but more commonly in the new Indian-
based religious movements which were springing up in the
fertile soil of student California: the Divine Light Mission,
Krishna Consciousness, and Transcendental Meditation.
Leary's colleague and co-conspirator, Richard Alpert,
renounced drugs, disappeared to India. and came back as a
guru with a new Hindu name, Ram Dass.

Yoga techniques of various kinds proliferated: *kundalini,
tantra, bhakti, raja.* But often there was little under-
standing of the underlying concepts; the glamour of the
East covered over a threadbare, naive philosophy. Gita
Mehta summed up the encounter of India and hippy
America:

> The seduction lay in the chaos. They thought they were
> simple. We thought they were neon. They thought we
> were profound. We knew we were provincial. Everybody
> thought everybody else was ridiculously exotic and
> everybody got it wrong.[11]

What, then, do the terms mean? What *are* the various
important forms of yoga? And what are the differences
between them? Let's begin to have a look.

---

[10] Gita Mehta, *Karma Cola* (London, 1981), p. 15.
[11] *Ibid.*, p. 5.

3
Hatha, Gnana, Karma, Bhakti, TM

When most people hear the word 'yoga', they mentally envisage someone sitting cross-legged on a mat doing exercises. Yoga can include much more than that, as we have already noticed – chanting *mantras,* meditating, ritual sex, experiments in magic – but most people think only of the exercise system. This is because *hatha* yoga (to give it its proper name) has become much more popular than any other type.

Hatha
The word *hatha* (pronounced 'hat-ha') is made up of the syllable *ha,* meaning 'moon', and *tha,* which means 'sun'. The reason for this is that yogis believe there are two warring currents, or impulses, set in motion every time we breathe – the 'moon' one (*prana vayu*) which begins in the area of the heart and ascends through the body up to the brain, and the 'sun' one (*apana vayu*) which starts around the solar plexus and heads downwards towards the anus. The discord created by the contrary pulls of these two currents is responsible for the continual restlessness we experience in body and mind. Therefore if it were possible to harness the 'sun' and 'moon' currents, and make them unite, the body and mind would be stilled, and we should be free to concentrate on our true Self.

This is exactly what *hatha* yoga tries to do. The exercises and breathing-techniques are all designed to create a situation in which the 'moon' current turns downwards, and the 'sun' current upwards, until they meet and lock together.

The upshot of this is that we have one united current of *prana* in our body, ready to be directed wherever we want it to go. (*Prana* is the vital life-energy which exists in all things, and which we breathe into our body every time we inhale.) What we should then do is push the concentration of energy down to the base of the spine. Here there is situated one of the seven *chakras* (spiritual energy centres) of the body, and also the entrance to the *sushumna*, the central spinal canal.

Now in most people the *sushumna* is never opened, as long as they live. But when a yogi manages to push *prana* into it, he suddenly finds that the spiritual life has become all at once much easier. For one thing, he can concentrate his mind much more readily, and so can go straight into stages 6, 7 and 8 of Patanjali's yoga ladder of progress. Alternatively, he can begin to awaken the *kundalini*, the strange and dangerous power which lies coiled at the base of the *sushumna*, and begin to experience *kundalini* yoga (an arcane variety, which we shall examine more fully in the next chapter). A whole range of spiritual options open themselves up to him.

This, then, is what the physical exercises are really for. (Actually, *hatha* includes three kinds of activity: the *asanas*, posture exercises; techniques of hygiene and cleansing, including rules about diet and fasting; and the *kumbhakas*, methods of breath control. It is really illegitimate to attempt one without the others.) As Hittleman states quite clearly, 'The health benefits...are actually by-products.'[1] Stephen Annett concurs: 'Although there is no well defined point at which [hatha] yoga merges into a higher discipline, and although yoga and keep-fit both concern themselves with the health of the body, the two are really poles apart.'[2]

Consequently there are widely differing attitudes expressed towards *hatha* by teachers of various schools. Some Indian sages have looked with distaste upon *hatha* yoga, believing that at best it is a series of preliminary exercises to be gone through before *real* yoga starts. Others have emphasized its importance; and the influential teacher B. K. S. Iyengar holds that the spiritual development of the Western world is at such a crude stage that the simplest basics of *hatha* yoga are all that the average Westerner can understand. But Christopher Isherwood believes that over-concentration upon it can be dangerous:

[1] R. L. Hittleman, *Yoga: The Eight Steps to Health and Peace*, p. 108.
[2] Stephen Annett, *The Many Ways of Being* (London, 1976), p. 91.

...it has been condemned by spiritual teachers because it tends, in practice, to concentrate the mind upon the body itself...it may be effective, certainly, but also dangerous. Over-indulgence in breathing exercises... may lead to hallucinations and, possibly, insanity. And, even at best, an excessive preoccupation with our physical appearance and well-being is obviously a distraction...[3]

Christians are more likely to be concerned about a different question: is it possible to divorce the (undoubtedly beneficial) exercise system from the elaborate Hindu theorizing about *sushumnas, prana* and *kundalini*? However little the gurus may like it, *is* it possible to practise *hatha* for health benefits alone, without taking on board the extra philosophical baggage appended to it? If so, then we can adopt the genuine insights and discard the rest; if not, there is nothing in *hatha* yoga for us.

This is a question we shall examine in chapter 5. Meanwhile, in passing, we should note clearly one fact: that if *hatha* yoga has anything to do with suppleness of the knees and relief from arthritis, it is really only by accident. Physical health is not its main concern.[4]

The British Wheel of Yoga concentrates heavily on *hatha* yoga, as might be expected, but tries to promulgate 'integral yoga', which includes *hatha* with four other types. We ought now to have a look at the other four. One of them (*raja*) we shall say more about in the next chapter; but what are *gnana* yoga, *karma* yoga and *bhakti* yoga?

Gnana
Gnana yoga is the yoga of wisdom and discrimination. It consists mainly of mental effort and is thought to be suitable for people of an intellectual cast of mind. It involves three main activities. One is meditation upon the Vedic scriptures; the second is a habit of thoughtful, discriminating

[3] Swami Prabhavananda and Christopher Isherwood, *How to Know God: The Yoga Aphorisms of Patanjali* (London, 1969), pp. 47–48.

[4] In fairness, however, it should be said that *in practice* physical fitness is the primary aim of many *hatha* adherents – in India as well as in the West.

analysis of all the occurrences and circumstances of life, with a view to discarding the distractions of *maya* and seeing right through to what is real and eternal beyond the surface of everyday events. But the ordinary, logical, reasoning mind cannot do this, and so the *gnana* yogi will reach the stage of frustration when he realizes that thought can take him no further. At this point of absolute despair the true Self will reveal itself to him – in incommunicable experience, not reasoned argument – and at last he will Know Absolutely. This is the third activity: the jettisoning of the logical mind in favour of direct experience. The scriptures compare the process to stirring a funeral pyre with a stick. At first, the stick is cold and separate from the fire; but eventually, by contact, it ignites and is finally consumed.

Karma

Karma yoga is the yoga of everyday life. Perhaps the best-known of the Indian scriptures, but one which we have not mentioned up till now, is the *Bhagavad-Gita,* a poem which celebrates a conversation between Krishna (one of the personal forms taken by God in order to communicate with men) and the warrior, Arjuna. Arjuna expresses his concern that the active life he leads is leaving him no time for spiritual development; what should he do? Krishna reveals to him that work can be worship; he should not seek total inactivity (which is impossible), but instead transform his work so that it becomes a form of devotion to Krishna.

Out of this idea has come *karma* yoga, the attitude of mind which attempts to take work seriously as a form of divine service, and not as a fulfilment of personal wants or desires. Work cannot be avoided, as Krishna stressed ('Verily, no one can remain, even for a moment, without doing work...everyone is made to act, in spite of himself'[5]), but it is important not to do it simply to satisfy our own cravings. If we do, we shall never attain the attitude of detachment from *maya* which all yoga is trying to achieve.

The best-known *karma* yogi of the twentieth century was probably Mahatma Gandhi, a man in whom an incredible

[5] *Bhagavad-Gita* III, 5.

work-rate was combined with an unrelenting spiritual thirst. 'Satisfaction should be sought in the work done,' he taught, 'not in its outcome.'[6] And: 'We do not decide what the results of our action will be; that is God's prerogative.'[7] What infuriated and fascinated Westerners, who worked with him, about Gandhi's attitude to work and politics was his curious air of being totally detached from the issues in which he was involved. It was not that he did not care deeply about his country or its future; but he was a difficult man to negotiate with, because there was a strange, almost impersonal, fatalistic objectivity in his approach to the problems of living. He was a *karma* yogi.

Perhaps because it is not so quiescent as the other forms, *karma* yoga has a long-standing connection with Indian political independence of mind. Another twentieth-century *karma* yogi was Sri Aurobindo, a brilliant, Cambridge-educated political administrator who received a year's imprisonment in 1908 for sedition and conspiracy. Although in prison he had a spiritual experience which led him to renounce his political involvement in favour of teaching yoga, he never lost his concern for changing the world and furthering human progress. Repeatedly he stressed that he was not interested in taking people out of the world through yoga, but in making them more effective within it; and he believed that humanity was in a transitional state, on its way to realizing the kingdom of heaven on earth by releasing its true Self and discovering its potential divinity. And so the Aurobindo type of yoga has definite material aims. This has been expressed since 1964 in the setting up of 'Auroville', a model town near Pondicherry in India, where the ideals of Aurobindo are to be worked out practically in an ideal community.

Aurobindo (who died in 1950 after twenty-four years under a vow of silence) has only a few followers in Britain, but is revered by many more, and his writings are extremely influential. He taught various forms of yoga, but emphasized that *karma* was the form best suited to our times.

[6] Mahatma Gandhi, *Ethical Religion* (Madras, 1924), p. 41.
[7] Quoted by Mahadev Desai, *Ghandiji in Indian Villages* (Madras, 1927), p. 86.

The International Society for Krishna Consciousness would dispute that claim. Nor would they accept that the *Bhagavad-Gita* is really about *karma* yoga. For ISKCON believes passionately in another type of yoga: *bhakti*.

Bhakti

Krishna devotees have become some of the best-known Indian cult followers in the Western world, because they are hard to miss. Dancing along the main shopping-streets, beating hand-drums and ringing cowbells, shaven-headed and swathed in saffron robes, the Krishna people are an unusual, colourful sight, though they often appear in ordinary Western dress. They have caught attention, too, by their up-to-date methods. At one stage a record of the Hare Krishna *mantra*, produced for them by George Harrison, penetrated the upper reaches of the pop charts, and more recently they developed a 'Palace on Wheels' – an incredible juggernaut lorry which combines a travelling exhibition, Krishna temple, and sacred food kitchen, and carries the message of Krishna Consciousness to market-places and country shows all over England.

Krishna Consciousness began with a young Indian businessman, Abhay Charan De, who in 1922 fell under the spell of a guru with the imposing title of His Divine Grace Sri Simad Bhakti Siddhanta Saraswati Goswami Prabhupada. De's guru reminded him of how some centuries earlier an Indian sage, the Lord Chaitanya, had started a joyful revivalist movement, based on chanting *mantras* to Krishna, among the poorer people in Indian towns and villages; and De began to conceive the idea of doing the same thing again, but this time throughout the entire world. The Prabhupada died in 1936, but two weeks before his death sent De a letter commanding him to fulfil his mission, and to do it through the medium of English.

De started slowly. It was 1944 before he began his now world-famous magazine, *Back to Godhead,* and 1947 before he acquired the title 'Bhaktivedanta' as a recognition of his eminence as a sage and teacher. In 1950 he began the process of becoming a *sannyasi,* someone completely detached from ordinary society, by leaving Calcutta to live

25

apart from his wife, sons and daughter. It cannot have been an easy step for a 58-year-old family man with a prosperous pharmaceutical business of his own.

Finally, by 1965, he decided the time had come to expand his activities to the Western world. He therefore travelled inconspicuously to New York, on a slow freighter, and when he arrived he simply sat down in Tomkins Park and started chanting. The sight of an aged Indian in yellow robes sitting under a tree and worshipping Krishna soon drew attention, and he started to make influential converts. Beat poet Allen Ginsberg became involved. English lecturer Howard Wheeler of Ohio State University changed his name to 'Hayagrivadas' and started chanting, too.

From there, the movement has spread world-wide. Swami Prabhupada (as De was known by the movement) arrived in America at a propitious moment, just as the drug craze was peaking, and young people were looking for spiritual answers in novel forms. But ISKCON has survived much better than most of the neo-Hindu groups of the sixties, simply because it demands so much of its followers. Prabhupada was a man of remorseless personal discipline, and he expected no less of any Krishna devotee. Consequently the tough, exhausting life-style of the movement will never attract millions of followers, but it *does* offer a challenge to the thoroughly determined, and anyone who lasts long enough to join the movement is unlikely to leave very quickly.

What does *bhakti* yoga teach? The word *bhakti* means 'devotion', and in this form of yoga the adherent is supposed to achieve union with ultimate reality by giving his love and worship unremittingly to one of the personal forms of God. (Confusingly, although *Brahman* is supposed to be an impersonal force, Hindus believe that the Godhead can also be worshipped as a person, under a whole variety of names.) One way of devoting oneself is to chant, over and over again, a sacred form of words, which will set up cosmic vibrations in the atmosphere around one's body and bring the power of the God addressed to bear upon one's life. This sacred form of words is called a *mantra,* and although there are thousands of them the Hare Krishnas are especially attached to one, the *Maha mantra*, or 'Great Hymn':

Hare Krishna, Hare Krishna,
Krishna Krishna, Hare Hare,
Hare Rama, Hare Rama,
Rama Rama, Hare Hare.

By chanting this incessantly, they believe, we lose attachment to material things, and are drawn away from the fascinations of *maya* to fall in love with reality itself. Faye Levine, a researcher who studied the Krishna Consciousness movement for some time, comments: 'I saw that chanting was crucial to the Hare Krishnas' state of mind. For starters, it regularized the breathing, drove out all other thoughts, helped you forget yourself, made you feel a part of the group, and filled up your head with itself.'[8] Whether this means a confrontation with ultimate reality, or a withdrawal into a make-believe world of emotional simplicity, is a matter of judgment.

Most *bhakti* yogis are monists, that is, they believe that God is ultimately impersonal, and that worshipping a personal form of God is just an effective way of getting to the impersonal essence; but not the Krishna people. For them, Krishna in a personal form is the ultimate, and *Brahman* is included in Krishna. Therefore devotion to Krishna is the highest and most important form of yoga; the others are at best only aids to it. In his book *The Perfection of Yoga* Swami Prabhupada claims that other forms of yoga practised in the West are incapable of bringing spiritual success in this degraded age:

At the utmost we can only gratify our personal whims by some pseudo-adaptation of this system. Thus people are paying money to attend some classes in gymnastic exercises and deep-breathing, and they're happy if they think they can lengthen their lifetimes by a few years or enjoy better sex life.... Such show-bottle performances have nothing to do with the actual perfection of yoga.

[8] Faye Levine, *The Strange World of the Hare Krishnas* (New York, 1974), p. 60.

The material disease cannot be cured by artificial medicine. We have to take the real cure straight from Krishna.[9]

TM

Another form of yoga which makes sizeable claims for itself, and ignores all the others, is TM, or Transcendental Meditation. The origins of it bear some similarity to the story of ISKCON: a Westernized Indian (in this case a physics graduate named Mahesh Prasad Warna) meets a spiritual teacher (Swami Brahmananda Saraswati) who becomes his guru and on his deathbed commissions the disciple to go to the West in order to enlighten it. The disciple changes his name (Prasad Warna is now Maharishi Mahesh Yogi) and comes to the West, initially in obscurity but eventually finding wide acclaim in the mid-sixties.

Maharishi, of course, became famous initially for the temporary influence he had over the Beatles. TM as a movement has always had the knack of attracting the famous and influential, probably because – unlike ISKCON – it plays down its religious origins as far as possible and presents itself as a neutral therapy which anyone can undertake without prejudice to his existing religious views.

This, however, is not the case, as anyone even slightly acquainted with the theory of yoga can plainly see; and as a result Maharishi has lost two important lawsuits in New Jersey which hung upon the question of whether TM was a religious movement or not. In fact, Maharishi's own books make it quite clear that TM is a Hindu yoga movement of a fairly recognizable traditional type.

In my own book about Maharishi,[10] I described him as a 'Hindu *bhakti* yogi'. This is not *quite* accurate, for although TM relies upon the *bhakti* yoga technique of chanting mantras, it is an 'impersonalist' movement which places no importance upon any particular personality of God. Not outwardly, anyway; there is some evidence to show that the

[9] A. C. Bhaktivedanta Swami Prabhupada, *The Perfection of Yoga* (London, 1972), pp. 28–29.

[10] John Allan, *TM: A Cosmic Confidence Trick* (Leicester, 1980), p. 16.

mantras given to meditators by Maharishi are all specific names of Hindu deities. R. D. Scott, who used to be a TM teacher, first started having doubts about the movement when he was given a new *mantra* which he managed to translate. It meant, 'Most beautiful Aiing, I bow down to you.' Aiing is the name of a Hindu creator god in the *Tantra Asana*.[11]

Maharishi himself admits that the purpose of the *mantra* is 'to produce an effect in some other world, to draw attention of those higher beings or gods living there. The entire knowledge of the mantra…is devoted to man's connection, to man's communication with the higher beings in a different strata (*sic*) of creation.'[12] In view of statements such as this, there is room for doubt as to whether TM is really as 'impersonalist' and non-devotional as in public it claims to be.

One of the most worrying features of TM practice – though not one of the most well-known – is the repeated incidence of phenomena, amongst advanced meditators, of the kind which Christians have traditionally seen as signs of demonic oppression. And the movement itself openly claims the ability to confer occult powers, such as clairvoyance, invisibility, levitation and astral travel. Just how much is occultism a feature of yoga practice? That is the question I want to examine in our next chapter.

4

Yoga and the paranormal

Yogis have always been vaguely connected with strange powers, in the Western mind. Indian rope-tricks, firewalking, lying on beds of nails – holy men of the East have a generally mystical reputation which some of them would like to lose. 'I have even been asked,' complains B. K. S. Iyengar, '…whether I can drink acid, chew glass, walk

[11] *Ibid.*, p. 35.
[12] *Meditations of Maharishi Mahesh Yogi* (New York, 1973), pp. 17–18.

through fire, make myself invisible or perform other magical arts.'[1] Gita Mehta tells of an ascetic in Rishikesh who lies outside a temple on a bed of nails and pieces of steel, with the following message written on a slate by his side:

> Yes, I am a sadhu. Yes, I have not spoken for twelve years. Yes, my body still feels some pain and some discomfort. Please leave me alone to meditate on the Universal Absolute.[2]

Where strange powers exist, in other words, they are not to be focused on for their own sake; like the health benefits of *hatha*, they are merely a by-product, and not at all the major goal; only the charlatan will try to make a reputation for himself out of them. Nonetheless, yoga has always involved some commerce with the occult and esoteric, and as far back as Patanjali the connection was acknowledged quite openly. The third part of the *Yoga Sutras* describes the occult powers (known as *siddhis*) which should result from an application of Patanjali's sixth, seventh and eighth stages of *raja* yoga: knowledge of the past and future; instinctive understanding of foreign languages and animal sounds; knowledge of one's past lives; invisibility; knowledge of the exact time of one's death; paranormal strength; psychic insight into the secrets of nature; visions of celestial beings; and much more, right up to 'omnipotence and omniscience'.

On the basis of Patanjali's claims, Swami Vivekananda taught that 'the yogi can enter a dead body and make it get up and move, even while he himself is working in another body. Or he can enter a living body, and hold that man's mind and organs in check, and for the time being act through the body of that man.'[3]

It is difficult to know how to assess claims like this. On the other hand, some outstanding feats of physical endurance have been achieved by yogis – as they have by Voodoo dancers in Haiti, witch-doctors in Central Africa

---

[1] B. K. S. Iyengar, *Light on Yoga*, p. 13.

[2] Gita Mehta, *Karma Cola*, p. 56.

[3] Quoted by Swami Prabhavananda and Christopher Isherwood, *How to Know God*, p. 131.

30

and *dang-kis* in the spiritualist cults of Singapore, all of whom have remarkably different outlooks on the nature of the world. On the other hand, for the more ambitious claims made by Patanjali, all we can say is that there is no hard evidence for the existence of such powers. Whenever a yoga group has claimed to be able to demonstrate them the results have been disappointing. TM, for example, asserts that it can teach people to levitate, and publishes pictures of meditators hovering in the air; but the movement will not allow levitation to be witnessed or filmed, since it was demonstrated that trained athletes could simulate the 'levitations' by a sudden downward muscular thrust of their legs against the floor.

Warnings against the occult
Western commentators are often embarrassed by the latent occultism of yoga, and sometimes suggest that it has no real application in our materialist society. Isherwood and Prabhavananda, for example, insist that:

> Western man...has preferred to concentrate on the production of mechanical rather than psychological powers; and so, instead of telepathy, we have the telephone, instead of levitation we have the helicopter, and instead of clairvoyance we have television... So let us stop hankering after the psychic powers and turn back to the true path toward spiritual growth...[4]

Some irresponsible Hindu-based groups make a great deal of capital out of the miracle-working abilities of their leader. But the *Sutras* warn that there are 'invisible beings in high places' who will use occult abilities as a snare to tempt the yogi from progressing further into the knowledge of reality; the true yogi should cultivate an air of detachment from them, and concentrate on advancing beyond them into a deeper experience of *Brahman*. Thus responsible yogis look with disfavour upon anyone who makes contact with occult forces an end in itself; Swami Sivananda, for instance, warns against spiritualism:

[4] *Ibid.*, p. 127.

The spirits have no knowledge of the highest truth. They cannot help others in attaining Self-realisation. Some are foolish, deceitful and ignorant...No-one should allow himself to become a medium. The mediums have lost the power of self-control. Their vital energy, life-force and intellectual powers are used by the spirits which control them. The mediums do not gain any higher divine knowledge.[5]

This comes remarkably close to the traditional Christian view of spiritualism and the spirit world. The Bible makes it quite plain that there are evil entities with debased aims which can interact with human beings in a personal way, and lead them on into spiritual chaos by holding out the lure of paranormal powers. The difference between the two approaches is that Christianity never sanctions for a second the cultivation of supernatural abilities – even as a passing stage on a spiritual pilgrimage. *All* congress with the demonic is perilous; at the very least the advanced yogi is laying himself open to tremendous temptations, and for every determined, disciplined 'saint' who has developed beyond this stage of yoga, there must be several thousand ordinary Indians who have become ensnared in superstition and obsessed with trivial magic as a result. ('I have got a matrimonium (*sic*) problem,' reads one letter to *Yoga Today,* 'and I like somebody is a powerful person to help me, who knows occult as well as Tantrika to fix things up.'[6] Like it or not, that is the way Indians as well as Westerners tend to see the yogi wonder-worker.)

Kundalini
Be that as it may, there are two varieties of yoga (apart from *raja*) which are especially associated with occult powers: *kundalini* and *tantra*. *Kundalini,* you may remember, is the word used to describe an immensely powerful energy force reckoned to lie, coiled and dormant, at the base of the spine. *Kundalini* yoga involves various techniques for awakening the energy force and making it

[5] 'Sivananda on Spiritualism', *Yoga Today* 5:11, p. 45.
[6] *Yoga Today* 6:10, p. 20.

rise slowly up the *sushumna* (spinal column). As it rises, it passes through each of the *chakras* (the seven psychic centres of the human body, with the highest one at the top of the skull), and as it contacts each *chakra* various psychic experiences take place. When eventually the practitioner becomes skilled enough to raise the *kundalini* to the utmost *chakra,* he receives the ability to perform miracles and gain liberation from *maya*.

One of the most influential *kundalini* teachers today (and the man behind Joseph Dippong, whose story we told in chapter 1) is Gopi Krishna. In his assessment, 'Kundalini is the key to the locked reservoir of highly potent psychic energy in man which is the biological mechanism responsible for genius, intellectual eminence, paranormal talent and experience of higher dimensions of consciousness.' Whether or not this is true, one thing is certain: the awakening of the *kundalini* (whatever it really is) does have explosive effects upon the personality of the yogi who tries it. *Kundalini* yoga can be dangerous, much more so than the other forms we have looked at so far.

Some influential twentieth-century occultists, such as Gurdjieff and his disciple Peter Ouspensky, were totally opposed to any attempt to awaken the *kundalini* and warned their followers against it. Other traditional yogis have also concluded that it is unsafe for most people in the Western world. And most of those who teach it surround their instruction with strict conditions: 'The teacher must be in superb physical, mental and spiritual health,' insists Dr Swami Gitananda, 'and the candidate purified by two to five years of rigid Hatha Yoga, Pranayama disciplines.'[7] One can see why, when reading the experiences of *kundalini* adepts such as Paramahansa Muktananda. For example:

> ...I felt severe pain in the knot (*manipur chakra*) below the navel. I tried to shout but could not even articulate. It seemed as if something was stuck in my throat. Next I saw ugly and dreadful demon-like figures. I thought them to be evil spirits.

[7] Quoted by Dr Swami Gitananda, 'Kundalini – Fact and Fiction', *Yoga Today* 6:10, p. 14.

I then saw blazes of fire on all sides and felt that I too was burning. After a while I felt a little better. Suddenly I saw a large ball of light approaching me from the front; as it approached, its light grew brighter and brighter. It then entered unobstructed through the closed doors of my *kutir* and merged into my head. My eyes were forcibly closed and I felt a fainting sensation.[8]

Tantrism

Most forms of yoga involve discipline and self-denial. But in the seventh century a group of texts were written which began to suggest the possibility of using some of the natural impulses of the body in yoga, rather than simply trying to suppress or ignore them. Sex, especially, was seen as a possible route to the experience of ultimate reality; in sexual intercourse there is a sense of merging of male and female, and the writers of these treatises argued that by prolonging the sex act, so as to deny the male climax entirely and enhance the female experience, it should be possible to set up a flow of sexual energy between the two partners that both began to experience the ultimate Oneness of the universe.

These treatises are known as the *Tantras,* and the form of yoga deriving from them is *tantric* yoga. Most orthodox Hindus regard it as a scandalous, libidinous excuse for excess; but in fact it involves very strict self-control of three factors: the breath, through various exercises; the mind, which must be stilled completely; and the seminal fluid, which must not be allowed to escape. In tantric sex the couple stand virtually motionless, the woman maintaining her partner's excitement (and her own) by skilful movements of the vaginal muscles. Anything less like an orgy it would be hard to imagine.

Tantrism had an impact on Buddhism, too, especially in Tibet, where the synthesis of life and death created as much interest as the synthesis of male and female. Tibetan Tantrism concerned itself with the after-death state, and produced a book known as the *Bardo Thodol* (loosely translated, 'Limbo Teachings'), or *Tibetan Book of the*

[8] Amma, *Swami Muktananda Paramahansa* (Ganeshpuri, 1971), p. 33.

Dead. The *Bardo Thodol* outlines the various stages of the death experience, and supplies *mantras* to assist meditation upon each stage. Thus the user can meditate upon death in the midst of life, and prepare himself for the journey he must some day undertake.

The point behind this is that after his death a priest or relative will intone some of the *mantras* for about fourteen days (in some cases, forty-nine). It is believed that the *mantras* will be perceived by the dead person, and his previous meditation will help him to recognize the various stages of death as they happen to him.

This is important, because without this recognition he will sink into a second death, and be more deeply immersed in *maya* than when he was alive. When reborn, he will still be enslaved to passions and blinded by the truth. But the tantric yogi 'comes into existence in the mother's womb knowingly, remains in it knowingly, and comes out of it knowingly',[9] and is thus able to wander at will, with unbroken continuity of consciousness, out of one life and into the next.

Life and death, male and female – the tantric attempt to find synthesis consists of dramatically forcing together obvious opposites. Not surprisingly, as a result it has caught the imagination of many power-seekers in the Western world, and tantric or pseudo-tantric groups are arousing a great deal of interest. The *Tantras* give a lot of attention to magic, spells and rituals, and the whiff of occultism over-hanging Tantra groups adds to their romantic appeal.

Some of the tantric teachers are extremely clever men. Professor Aghenanda Bharati, for instance, an Italian anthropologist, became a convert to tantric ideas as a result of encountering what he calls the 'zero-experience': the sensation of absolute oneness with the universe, and loss of personal identity.[10] Interestingly, he refuses to believe the claims of traditional gurus that they can live in a permanent state of 'zero-experience'; he claims to have had the sensation only six times himself, sometimes as a result of tantric sexual practices.

[9] 'Samgiti Sutta', Pali Canon.
[10] Aghenanda Bharati, *The Light at the Centre* (Santa Barbara, 1976).

The 'Orange People'

Much better known is US-based ex-philosophy professor Bhagwan Shree Rajneesh, whose disciples attract publicity by their flamboyance and sheer permissiveness of life-style. When someone joins the movement, a new name is given, and there is a requirement always to wear orange clothing and carry a picture of Rajneesh; but apart from that, rules are at a minimum. 'Just by living totally in the world,' Bhagwan teaches, 'you will transcend it.'

> The old sannyas said: Escape, renounce.
> But I tell you, those who escape are not total, not whole,
> I tell you that those who escape are crippled.
> It is not for you.
> You live life in its totality
> You live life as wholly as possible
> And the more whole you are
> the more holy you will become.[11]

Living life in its totality can bring notoriety. At least one of Bhagwan's female followers, Ma Prem Hamida, has appeared as a pin-up in the 'girlie' magazine *Mayfair*, dressed – almost – in the famous orange clothing. At Easter 1981 a mass sex-therapy course in London attracted such headlines as LOVE-IN AT THE CAFE ROYAL and THE SEXY GURU AND HIS MESSAGE OF FREE LOVE. The 'Orange People' are unabashed: most human hang-ups, they say, come from sex, and learning to respond to it naturally and unashamedly brings integration, wholeness and spiritual power.

Rajneesh denies being a follower of any particular path ('I am the beginning of a tradition, not the end...I have been like a bee going from one flower to another, gathering many fragrances'[12]), but he undeniably fits into the 'tantric' pigeon-hole more readily than any other. His form of meditation involves violent movement, chaotic breathing, shaking the body; this produces a state of euphoria, which his followers claim to be enlightenment. 'A sort of quiet

[11] Brochure for Kalptaru Meditation Centre (London), distributed in 1980.
[12] *Ibid.*

hysteria sets in,' complains Charles Lovell, of the British Wheel of Yoga, 'when imprinting of dogma and life style can take place.'[13]

Certainly Rajneesh attracts dog-like, uncritical devotion from his admirers, and there is some irony in the sign which used to stand outside the lecture-hall in his Poona headquarters: 'Shoes and Minds are to be left here at the gate.' The mind is our enemy, according to Bhagwan, 'the chatterbox in your head that you cannot switch off'. 'The mind is so subtle – it can deceive you, it can make you feel that you are a great seeker because you are asking, "What is God?", "Who created the world?", "Why are we here?", "What is the purpose of life?", and all these questions are stupid.'[14]

Traditional yoga certainly teaches that the mind needs to be transcended, but not that it needs to be thrown away. Yet for the 'Orange People' that is the price of enlightenment, and what Bhagwan offers is an unthinking, unevaluated emotional trip which aims at gratifying rather than sublimating the personal desires of the adherent. Loss of individuality is not the goal; he teaches that, with each spiritual advance, the ego simply becomes more subtle. It does not die away, as in most forms of yoga; rather it becomes stronger.

Other Tantra groups

There are several other important Tantra groups. There is *Ananda Marga,* for one, formed in the 1950s to double as a tantric yoga teaching organization *and* a social action group ('Meditation is of little use to starving children'). There is the Scandinavian School of Yoga, whose tantric yoga classes are more thorough and less eccentric than anything else mentioned in this section so far. But best known of the remainder is the '3HO Foundation', organized by Yogi Bhajan, who claims somewhat immodestly to be the only teacher of tantric yoga in the world.

[13] Charles Lovell (reviewing *Meditation – the Art of Ecstasy* by Bhagwan Shree Rajneesh), *The Christian Parapsychologist* 3:8 (Sept. 1980), p. 286.

[14] Bhagwan Shree Rajneesh, *The White Lotus* (Poona, 1981), quoted in Rajneesh books catalogue.

'3HO' stands for 'healthy, happy and holy', and the main way in which the movement attempts to achieve these goals is the teaching of *kundalini* yoga. But tantric yoga can be taught, too – though only when Yogi Bhajan is personally present. 3HO's version of tantric yoga is less Sunday-tabloid material than that of other groups; couples are directed to adopt certain positions (*mudras*) and then sit and look at one another, while Yogi Bhajan directs operations and 'channels the energy'.

The 3HO Foundation is somewhat unusual in being a Sikh group, demanding that acolytes wear traditional Sikh dress and obey the rules for diet and life-style which Sikhs have always upheld. But then yoga has not for centuries been a purely Hindu practice. Traces of yoga will be found within Islam, Mahayana Buddhism, Taoism, Japanese Buddhism and Jainism. The question we must now examine is: could it be transferable into Christianity?

5
Is 'Christian yoga' possible?

If we want to understand how yoga and Christianity relate to one another, perhaps the first thing to do is to look at how yoga has come from Hinduism and become part of the other two leading world religions: Buddhism and Islam.

Yoga and Buddhism
The key to Buddhism is the word 'independence'. Buddhists are looking for the same kind of liberation from material *maya* as Hindus are; the difference is that, while Hinduism finds room to talk about the grace of God and the efficacy of following a guru, in Buddhism man is completely on his own. 'Look within,' proclaimed Lord Gautama, the founder of Buddhism, 'thou art the Buddha.' He showed an unwillingness to lay down precise rules for his followers ('Whoever wishes may dwell in the forest and whoever wishes may dwell in a village') and was often confusingly undogmatic about matters of belief:

Believe nothing just because you have been told it, or it is commonly believed, or because it is traditional or because you yourselves have imagined it. Do not believe what your Teacher tells you merely out of respect for the Teacher. But whatsoever, after due examination and analysis, you find to be conducive to the good, and benefit the welfare of all beings – that doctrine believe and cling to, and take as your guide.[1]

Experience is the arbiter of everything. Traditional authority can be a dangerous enemy of liberation, rather than a helpful guide; modern Zen master D. T. Suzuki admits, 'Anything that has the semblance of an external authority is rejected by Zen...Zen wants absolute freedom, even from God.'[2]

As might be expected, the pursuit of 'absolute freedom' has divided world Buddhism into a wide variety of emphases and approaches. Almost from the start, there was a deep philosophical split between the *Mahayana* (Great Vehicle) school, out of which has come Zen and Tantric Buddhism, and the *Theravada* (Way of the Ancients) school, stricter and more conservative. But in all forms of Buddhism the ultimate objective is the same: liberation from suffering through the extinction of material desire. Gautama taught that all life involves suffering, and the reason that we suffer is that we experience the frustration of our desires. If these natural desires could be burnt out, then we would suffer no longer.

Buddhism, then, is a practical guide to ways of living which will lead us out of slavery to desire. It is not a religion which focuses attention on the worship of a Supreme Being; Gautama's attitude was that, if the gods did exist, they were irrelevant anyway, since they were certainly not going to help. 'If indifference to a personal creator is atheism,' remarked Huston Smith, 'Buddha was indeed an atheist.'[3]

Gautama was born into a Hindu family, and the world-

[1] Quoted by Cris Popenoe, *Inner Development*, p. 147.
[2] D. T. Suzuki, *An Introduction to Zen Buddhism* (New York, 1964), pp. 44, 97.
[3] Huston Smith, *The Religions of Man* (New York, 1958), p. 112.

view of Buddhism comes very close to that of Hinduism. Life is cyclic, each man undergoing repeated incarnations. The material world is a place of illusion, pain and distraction. Enlightenment and ultimate release come from within. And so it is not surprising that Buddhism is prepared to make use of yoga as a spiritual practice *en route* to its version of liberation (*Nirvana*) – if only as a 'valuable, though less central, method of development'.[4] Buddhist Scriptures detailing paths to enlightenment cheerfully borrow yoga methods from Hinduism as an integral part of their recommendations:

> Then, my friend, you should find yourself a living-place which, to be suitable for Yoga, must be without noise and without people...Sitting cross-legged in some solitary spot, hold your body straight, and for a time keep your attention in front of you, either on the tip of the nose or the space on your forehead between the eyebrows. Then force your wandering mind to become wholly occupied with one object...[5]

Yoga and Sufism

Yoga's penetration into Islam has not been quite so complete. Most Muslims would have no use for it, but there is a body of mystics on the fringe of Islam called Sufis, to whom yoga practices are an acceptable part of faith. 'Sufi' means 'wearer of wool', and the sect began with a group of Arabian teachers among whom the wearing of wool was a mark of sanctity. Another possible origin of the name, according to modern Sufi writer Idries Shah, was that the word 'Sufi' 'contains, in enciphered form, the concept of Love'.

Love was important to the Sufis. Unlike other Muslims, who held that God was merciful to mankind but not a lover of individual men, they believed that it was possible to enter into an estatic love relationship with God, not unlike Patanjali's eighth stage, *samadhi*. (In fact modern Sufis will use this term quite freely: Pir Vilayat Inayat Khan, head of

[4] Catalogue of the London Buddhist Centre, issued 1981.

[5] Ashvaghosha, *Buddhacarita* II, tr. Edward Conze, in *Buddhist Scriptures*, ed. E. Conze (Harmondsworth, 1959).

the Sufi Order, has published a lecture on 'Samadhi in everyday life'.)

The Sufis existed precariously within Islam. Their mystical experiences ran so much counter to the received ideas of Islamic thought that they had to resort to cryptic devices in order to survive within the orthodox community: teaching in mystical symbols, rather than straightforward language; occasionally pretending to be mad; subscribing to the orthodox creed but giving it a personal interpretation:

> Provided that a person could assert that he subscribed ... he could not be proceeded against for heresy ... there was nothing in the phrase of affirmation which could not be subscribed to by a Sufi. His interpretation might be more mystical than that of the scholastics, but no power existed ... which could finally establish the ascendancy of the clerics.[6]

Because of the caution they had to exercise, it is often difficult to work out the plain meaning of what they were trying to say. Abu Yazid al-Bistami, who was expelled seven times from his native town but otherwise managed to avoid major persecution, seems to have taught that the Sufi who experiences God mystically merges into him and becomes one with him – very like a Hindu 'saint' merging with Brahman:

> I sloughed off my self as a snake sloughs off its skin, and I looked into my essence and saw that "I am He".[7]

If this were taken literally, it would be absolute blasphemy within the religion in which there is no God but one, and Muhammad is his prophet; and later thinkers qualified it. Junayd of Baghdad, for instance, agreed that in ecstasy the self and God seem to blend into one another, but claims that this is just 'the first isolation' of the soul, a trap which God sets for those who are spiritually proud. To become fascinated with this stage is wrong. One can push on beyond

[6] Idries Shah, *The Sufis* (London, 1977), p. 31.
[7] Quoted in R. C. Zaehner, *Hindu and Muslim Mysticism*, p. 186.

it into an I-Thou relationship with God in which one starts to see him as a separate entity once again.

All the same, it is clear that the Sufis are mutinously trying to import into Islam an experience very close to the ultimate goal of yoga. ('It is an odd paradox', remarks R. C. Zaehner, 'that Sufism, whose major premiss is the absolute distinction between man and God, should arrive at a conception of mystical experience that seems to be identical with that of the monistic Hindus who start from the totally contrary premiss that man is in some sense God.'[8]) And so it is no surprise that yoga methods and techniques should be appropriated by the Sufis in their search for *hagegut,* the abolition of earthly desires.

In the West today Sufism is spreading, and mainly amongst non-Islamic people. Writers such as Idries Shah, a cult figure especially in America, and younger leaders such as Inayat Khan have stressed that Sufism is not simply an Islamic cult, but a way of seeing the world which can be synthesized with many different religious outlooks. Inayat Khan in particular is a respected speaker on many 'New Age' platforms. (The 'New Age' movement is an amalgam of groups of all sorts of spiritual emphases who believe that we are witnessing the dawn of a great new era of spiritual diversity and power, the Aquarian Age. Inayat Khan is happy for Sufism to be part of the movement: '"Together we are one" is the slogan of the New Age,'[9] he observes.)

Beshara, an influential British Sufi group, makes a distinction between two types of Sufism: the traditional Islamic variety, which is a form of Islam, and 'real' Sufism, which they see as an esoteric tradition untied to any particular religion. They are adherents of the second variety: 'The man of wisdom,' they claim, 'whatever may happen, will never allow himself to be caught up in any one definite form or belief because he is wise unto himself.'[10] Beshara practices include some which bear similarities to yoga – the

[8] *Ibid.,* p. 14.

[9] Pir Vilayat Inayat Khan, 'Launching into the New Age', lecture published as part of booklet *Samadhi in Everyday Life* (Bradford-on-Avon, 1981).

[10] Beshara brochure, issued 1980.

42

chanting of Arabic names for God, for instance; forms of meditation; and breathing techniques.

Conclusions

What conclusions can we draw, then, about the place of yoga in religions outside Hinduism? The one into which it has slotted with no problems is Buddhism, and there are obvious reasons why this should be so: the similar world-view, philosophy and ultimate aims. Buddhism may now be a major world religion in its own right, but it began life as an extremely brilliant personal slant on Hinduism, originated by a Hindu.

The case of Islam presents more problems. To synthesize yoga with a religious system in which God is personal, not identical with man's true Self but distinct from it, the Sufis had to adopt an extremely symbolic, non-literal interpretation of the claims of the Koran. And the deeper they went in their mystical experiences, the more they left behind the orthodox Muslim view of God's personality, and the more they began to talk in terms of merging into God. God started to be seen less as a real, separate Person than as a force to be encountered in the depths of one's being.

What about Christianity? The Christian world-view (as we shall see in the next chapter) has very little in common with Hinduism or Buddhism. But it *does* share with Islam the conviction that God is a Person, who can be encountered in a personal way; and this suggests that there will be problems in trying to bring a yogic understanding into Christianity too. It may be possible, if we are vague enough about what Christian claims actually *mean* – just as the Sufis were with Islam; but if we take the plain statements of the Bible at face value, we may find contradictions which it is impossible to reconcile.

'All religions include yoga'

Writers who have discussed the relationship of Christianity and yoga have generally adopted one of six different positions. The first is that *all religions naturally include yoga anyway*. Christopher Isherwood remarks, 'There is no doubt that the great majority of believers, in all the world's

43

major religions, are fundamentally bhakti yogis.'[11] But he also identifies *karma* yoga in Christianity (St Vincent de Paul) and *gnana* yoga too (Thomas Aquinas). Even more sweepingly, an article in *Yoga Today* asserts, 'Every human being is, consciously or sub-consciously, living out a form of Yoga – finding his own approach to a gateway to the Divine within him.'[12]

But this is to use the term 'yoga' so broadly that it hardly means anything distinctive any more. *Bhakti* yoga, as we have seen, is an attempt to realize the true Self by giving oneself in devotion to a chosen divine figure – any divine figure. The aim of it is to escape the cycle of birth and death next time round. And this is such a long way from the motives behind Christian devotion to God, that to label it '*bhakti* yoga' is ridiculous.

For one thing, Christian love of God is not concerned with locating any 'true Self' hidden behind the veil of *maya*. Physical reality is not an illusion, but the good creation of a loving Father; 'everything created by God is good, and nothing is to be rejected if it is received with thanksgiving'[13] – not spurned and negated in the interests of spirituality. Furthermore, there can be no choice of divine figures to worship. The Bible claims that Jesus is not just *a* representation of God in human form, but *the* visible likeness of the invisible God.[14] His rank is far above any other being in the heavenly hierarchy:

> He reflects the glory of God and bears the very stamp of his nature, upholding the universe by his word of power ...For to what angel did God ever say, 'Thou art my Son, today I have begotten thee'?[15]

The early Christians were quite unabashed about this. 'There is salvation in no one else,' they insisted, 'for there is no other name under heaven given among men by which we

[11] Swami Prabhavananda and Christopher Isherwood, *How to Know God: The Yoga Aphorisms of Patanjali*, p. 107.

[12] Sri Balmukund Parikh and Elizabeth Fennell, 'The Ashram in Yoga', *Yoga Today* 5:7, p. 37

[13] 1 Timothy 4:4.   [14] Colossians 1:15.   [15] Hebrews 1:3, 5.

must be saved.'[16] I remember once talking to a Hare Krishna missionary on the street corner after buying a magazine from him. He was extremely keen to convert me until he found I was a Christian; at which he simply said, 'Oh well, you have your route, I have a better one,' and walked away to talk to someone else. To him, Krishna was simply the best route to deliverance, but my route would do; to me, as a Christian, Jesus is unique and Krishna is no substitute.

Again, as we shall see in the next chapter, the Christian hope is quite unconcerned with escaping the cycle of birth and death. To the Bible, there is no such thing as reincarnation: 'It is appointed for men to die once, and after that comes judgment.'[17] It is often claimed by yoga adherents who know a little bit of church history that Christian thinkers toyed with the idea of reincarnation for the first five centuries of the church's life, but that the idea was then rejected by the hard-line dogmatic theologians. Not so! Right from the start, the speculative Gnostic groups who theorized about reincarnation were seen as heretical by the Christian church, and some of the New Testament letters were written specifically to discredit their ideas. It is obvious from reading such books as 1 Thessalonians or 2 Peter that the real hope of the early Christians was the second coming of Jesus – an event for which they had only one lifetime to prepare.

'The lost secret of Christianity'
The second viewpoint on yoga and Christianity is that *yoga is really the lost secret of Christianity*. Maharishi Mahesh Yogi claims that world religion is in a mess because it has forgotten the technique of Transcendental Meditation:

> We need not describe in detail the deplorable state of religion in the world today...Only the rituals and dogma are found: the spirit has departed. That is why the followers of religion do not find fulfilment.[18]

[16] Acts 4:12.   [17] Hebrews 9:27.
[18] Maharishi Mahesh Yogi, *The Science of Being and Art of Living* (London, 1966), p. 256.

45

But TM holds the key. 'Here in a simple practice is the fulfilment of every religion...It existed in the early days of every faith and has since been lost.'[19] And other teachers of yoga make similar claims for other varieties of it. Looking at the history of religion, Swami Vivekananda asserted, 'Wherever there was any manifestation of what is ordinarily called supernatural power or wisdom, there a little current of kundalini must have found its way into the sushumna... All worship, consciously or unconsciously, leads to this end...What, thus, man ignorantly worships under various names, through fear and tribulation, the yogi declares to the world to be the real power coiled up in every being... yoga is the science of religion.'[20]

What are we to say to these claims? First, that although Christianity may seem to be 'losing its power' in the secularized West, this is by no means the case throughout the world. Although until recently it was thought that world Christianity had waned in numbers and influence since the start of the twentieth century, it is now known that the church is growing faster than ever it has before in history. Much of this growth is in countries where Christianity has made no impact until now; but even in the West, there are signs that Christian faith is making a come-back. Church attendance has reached an unusually high level in the USA, while in Britain it appears to be holding its own. Dead and meaningless religion indubitably exists, in many places; but it does not appear to have a monopoly.[21]

Second, Christians do not worship 'ignorantly...through fear and tribulation'. Genuine Christianity involves an open, free, daring relationship with a God who becomes a Father, a known and loved personality with whom friendship is possible:

[19] *Ibid.*, p. 259.
[20] Quoted in Prabhavananda and Isherwood, *How to Know God*, pp. 115–116.
[21] Figures on the growth of the Christian church world-wide are researched by the Missions Advanced Research Centre, Monrovia, California.

For you did not receive the spirit of slavery to fall back into fear, but you have received the spirit of sonship.[22]

Let us then with confidence draw near to the throne of grace, that we may receive mercy and find grace to help in time of need.[23]

Paul found in Athens a group of people who worshipped all sorts of gods, but had also built an altar 'To an unknown god', as they had a glimmering awareness that behind the multitude of religious hypotheses they had adopted there was still an unexplained element – a supreme power of overarching authority, whose name and nature they did not know. Paul sought to explain the 'unknown god' to them.

The God who made the world and everything in it, being Lord of heaven and earth, does not live in shrines made by man, nor is he served by human hands, as though he needed anything, since he himself gives to all men life and breath and everything.[24]

Vivekananda describes the God who lies behind the multitudinous forms of worship as impersonal, man-centred, *kundalini*; Paul describes him as personal, distinct from humanity, with a creative mind and will of his own. Once again, yoga's outlook on life clashes irreconcilably with the Bible's.

'Alter the objects of worship'

The third possible attitude need not detain us long, in view of what we have already said. It is that *yoga philosophy can be subsumed into Christianity by altering the objects of worship*. For example, J. Herbert, in his *Spiritualité hindoue,* declares: 'It must not be thought that the practices of the great yogis are inseparably tied to the concepts peculiar to Hindu theology...Nothing is simpler than to supply Western Christian names in place of Hindu in the treatises on Yoga technique.'[25] He suggests that in place of

---

[22] Romans 8:15.   [23] Hebrews 4:16.   [24] Acts 17:23–25.

[25] J. Herbert, *Spiritualité hindoue* (Paris, 1944), quoted by Jean-Marie Déchanet, *Christian Yoga* (London, 1965), p. 55.

Brahman we should read 'God the Father', in place of Rama 'Christ', in place of the goddess Kali 'Mary'.

But the problem is not as simple as that. It is a matter not of different names, but of different philosophies. 'Christianizing' yoga in this fashion is simply sweeping the problem under the carpet; and Jean-Marie Déchanet, a Christian monk who *is* involved in yoga, rightly brands Herbert's attitude as 'chicanery' and 'subterfuge'.

Dr Paul Brunton is one of the English popularizers most responsible for the spread of yoga in Britain earlier this century. He believes that Jesus instructed his personal followers in yoga and mysticism, and that the later apostles also became adepts ('there is ample evidence...such as in the mystic trances of John and the mystical sentences of Paul'). The New Testament contains a number of statements which must be read mystically, as referring to various yoga practices:

> The sentence 'the kingdom of heaven is within you' has absolutely no connection whatever with official religion and entirely refers to the experiences of yogis and mystics ...the compilation of these records in a single volume did not occur until a few hundred years after Jesus is believed to have passed away. The obscure Council of Nicea found numerous gospels extant when it sat to make the compilation, consisting of a mixed collection of religious books intended for the masses and mystical ones intended for the elect few...Hence the somewhat uneven selection...[26]

All one can say is that this sounds scholarly, but is entirely false. The first of the Gospels must have been written within a generation of Jesus' death, perhaps about fifteen years after, and all of the Gospels were in existence by the end of the first century. There was nothing 'obscure' about the Council of Nicea, and its job was not 'compilation' of anything. It simply met to recognize which books the church *had already*, throughout its history, recognized as authori-

[26] Paul Brunton, *The Hidden Teaching Beyond Yoga* (London, 1969), p. 65.

tative. And as far as life-stories of Jesus were concerned, there was no argument; the four Gospels had been long recognized as the only real accounts, and had been jealously safeguarded from any tampering.[27] There is no uneven jumbling of the 'religious' and the 'mystical'; the statement Brunton quotes about 'the kingdom of heaven' makes perfect sense in the passage in which it occurs, and the context shows that it has nothing whatsoever to do with yoga.

What Brunton is doing is trying to make bricks without straw. There is no evidence of any kind, anywhere, that Jesus ever taught anyone anything remotely resembling a yoga tenet or technique. The heart of his message had nothing to do with awakening the *kundalini*; more of this later.

'Yoga is an applied philosophy'

A fourth possible attitude is exemplified by Justin O'Brien's curious book, *Yoga and Christianity*. O'Brien is director of graduate studies at the Himalayan Institute of Pennsylvania, and, judging by both his name and his writing, a Catholic by upbringing. His view is that *yoga is an applied philosophy, not a religious system,* and therefore that seeming contradictions between yoga's viewpoint and Christianity's are apparent, not real. To compare the two is like comparing science and literature; they serve completely different ends. Christian doctrine is concerned with objective fact, questions of 'What?'; yoga is concerned with practical living, questions of 'How?'.

It sounds quite plausible until O'Brien tries to work it out; and then, alas, we encounter problems. For one thing, to force his system upon the Bible he has to fall back on the theory that there are different levels of meaning in the Bible, and so what seems to be a plain, literal statement may be anything but:

The complex truths of scriptures reveal a realm of reality, exceedingly intelligible, but disclosed by neither the

[27] See Xavier Léon-Dufour, *The Gospels and the Jesus of History*, tr. J. McHugh (London, 1968).

senses nor discursive reason. The normal faculties for contacting the world at large are limited when it comes to the apprehension of divine truths.[28]

To treat the Bible in this mystical way is to ignore the fact that it is not one book, but sixty-six, and large parts of it do make exceedingly plain and direct statements, which are patently intended to be taken literally. But insisting that anything we encounter could be symbolic has two benefits for O'Brien: first, he can dispense with the literal meaning of any statement which does not fit into his scheme; and second, he can present yoga as the real key to understanding Scripture:

> The type of exegesis that allows for the final resolution of biblical symbol is direct participation in the reality symbolized. The kingdom being within, one enters within to discover it... Inspired, literally filled with the spirit, all modes and degrees of the scriptural meanings become transparent... Like John on the island of Patmos, one has only to enter into his own spirit to reveal the cosmic mystery and fathom the Bible.[29]

This is playing fast and loose with what the Bible means when it says, 'Be filled with the Spirit.' The New Testament makes a clear distinction between the *human* spirit and the *Holy* Spirit, who is God, and who is necessary for us to achieve any degree of spiritual enlightenment. Understanding does not come by delving into the depths of our own human spirit, via yoga or anything else, but by opening up our lives to the presence and reality of the Holy Spirit, who is external to us:

> For all who are led by the Spirit of God are sons of God... When we cry, 'Abba! Father!' it is the Spirit himself bearing witness *with our spirit* that we are children of God.[30]

[28] Justin O'Brien, *Yoga and Christianity* (Honesdale, Pa., 1978), p. 17.
[29] *Ibid.*, p. 21.   [30] Romans 8:14–16 (my italics).

50

Thus, in order to synthesize Christianity and yoga, O'Brien has to sacrifice some important aspects of Christianity. Most important of all, Jesus starts to lose his uniqueness. O'Brien hints at this only obliquely, but it is obvious that he would like to see Jesus as no more than a souped-up human, a great example who could be emulated or even surpassed:

> Although Jesus manifested the same basic nature as others of the human race, the quality of his human expression sets him apart radically. No one would doubt his human competence. But whether theologians are justified in maintaining that Jesus' level of humanness is inaccessible to the rest of humanity...requires more evidence than is generally found in theological manuals.[31]

Christians, however, do not believe that Jesus was different from us because of 'the quality of his human expression'. He was different because he was God – a difference of kind, not just of degree. But O'Brien's watered-down Jesus is quite logical, if Jesus was no more than a master of yoga. Why should he be more important than a master of yoga in India, Tibet, or Japan? If his message was the same as theirs, why talk about uniqueness?

O'Brien's twists and turns demonstrate clearly that yoga is not simply an 'applied philosophy'. Like it or not, there are religious presuppositions built into the system, which will not allow us to absorb it into Christianity whole. The only other solution might be to dismantle the system, and try to select those bits which *can* be absorbed. This brings us to the fifth possible attitude: that of Jean-Marie Déchanet.

'Yoga as an aid to spiritual development'

Jean-Marie Déchanet is a French Benedictine monk who has been what he calls a 'yogi of Christ' for several years. His two books, *Christian Yoga* and the much more eccentric *Yoga and God*,[32] are probably the best-known works on yoga from a Christian standpoint, and have inspired many

[31] J. O'Brien, *op. cit.*, p. 61.
[32] London, 1965 and 1974 respectively. Tr. Roland Hindmarsh.

Christians to make forays into yoga for themselves. Permissible yoga, to him, is basically *hatha* yoga (although in his second book he does deal with *kundalini* yoga too), and he sees clearly that it must be divorced from its Hindu origins if it is to be useful to a Christian.

> It was essential that my exercises should turn me not towards the Self, the It, the Absolute, the Wholly-One, the vague 'ungraspable' of Hindu mystics, but towards the God of Abraham, Isaac and Jacob, the living God, Three in One, the principle of all things, my Creator and Father, him in whom I had natural and supernatural life. I felt it was absolutely necessary that my experiment should place itself under the protection and sanction of grace.[33]

Déchanet is not primarily concerned with the health-giving benefits of yoga, though he recognizes that those exist, His major concern is to use yoga as an aid to spiritual development. It is not the secret of living the Christian life, nor the power behind it; but it can make the service of God that bit easier:

> Every day the exercises, and indeed the whole ascetic discipline of my Yoga, make it easier for the grace of Christ to flow in me. I feel my hunger for God growing, and my thirst for righteousness, and my desire to be a Christian in the full strength of the word – to be for Christ, to be of Christ, without any half-measures or reservations.[34]

The difference between Christian yoga and traditional yoga is that the latter meant 'an absolute turning inwards on oneself...an absolute silence of the mind that shuts itself off from any outside influence, even though this should be divine...a mysticism lacking both dogma and faith'.[35] Christian yoga is simply a preparation for communion with Another, an emptying of oneself in order to appreciate

[33] J.-M. Déchanet, *Christian Yoga*, pp. 3-4.
[34] *Ibid.*, p. 13.   [35] *Ibid.*, pp. 15–16.

more fully the grace of God. The goal of it should not be altered states of consciousness, detachment from the material world, or contact with an imaginary 'true Self'; but simply an increased ability to enjoy God and serve him with unmixed motives.

It will be obvious that this is a much more careful, self-consistent position than any of those we have examined so far. Personally I have a great deal of sympathy for it. But there are a few questions which must be asked.

First, it is obvious that Déchanet is a thoughtful and sophisticated theologian. It may be possible for him to do the intellectual demolition job necessary to clear away the usual philosophical trappings of yoga, and erect instead a Christian system in its place; but what about the ordinary Christian without Déchanet's grounding in both Christian theology and Eastern thought? Would he be able to follow the Christian yogi along the tightrope (to change the metaphor) without overbalancing and falling off?

Second, just how important can yoga be in spiritual development? If it were of such massive value as Déchanet asserts, would one not expect to find at least *something* similar to it in the practice of Jesus or the apostles? Does the absence of anything like it from the New Testament not suggest that it is likely to be a very peripheral activity indeed?

Third, what is actually happening in *hatha* yoga? If we dismiss the Hindu theorizing about the *sushumna* and the twin currents of *prana* – theorizing for which no scientific evidence exists or is sought – where do the benefits of yoga actually come from? It may be objected that it scarcely matters, as long as it works; fair enough. But our ignorance of *why* it works prevents us from asking, 'Would something else work equally well? And are its results *all* positive?'

That raises a fourth question. Déchanet sees that the search for the true Self is unchristian and has no place in Christian yoga. Yet the techniques of *hatha* yoga have evolved with this aim in view, and they work to produce in us experiences which reinforce the idea that we *do* have another Self which is eternal and identifiable with God. Is it possible that the practice of *hatha* yoga will subtly alter one's view of reality in a monistic direction? There are worrying signs in Déchanet's second book that he has lost some of the balance he so impressively exhibited in the first. Will the practice of yoga in fact increase one's hunger for God, or will it simply expose one to the risk of increasing self-absorption?

Finally, *hatha* yoga was not really designed to stand on its own, as an independent system. Its practice was supposed to create a level of self-integration which would make it possible to advance to *raja* yoga or to the controlling of the *kundalini*. Will it in fact lead as readily into Christian spirituality? Or will the type of experiences it engenders create instead the sort of hunger which can only be fed by yoga experiments of a much less neutral type?

'A gateway into the occult'

There are answers to all of these questions; but no easy ones. Unless, that is, we opt for the sixth possible attitude to Christianity's relationship with yoga: that *yoga is a gateway into the occult, and so can produce demonic results.*

This has been the typical response of many Evangelicals to this subject. In many Christian paperbacks, yoga is lumped together with witchcraft, ouija, horoscopes, crystal balls and spiritualism as a means whereby the devil can gain control of a human life. Is this fair?

The Bible does teach quite plainly that there is a realm of spiritual reality inhabited by forces which are inimical to human beings. 'We are not contending against flesh and blood,' writes the apostle Paul, 'but...against the world rulers of this present darkness, against the spiritual hosts of wickedness in the heavenly places.'[36] It is possible for these forces, which are personal just as God is, to inhabit a human life in order to distract and destroy it; and such things as magic, sorcery and contacting the dead, specifically warned against in Scripture, are activities which can encourage this invasion by evil forces.

Now it is obvious, from our earlier description, that there are types of yoga which are playing about with magic. Tantric yoga is one, and I have personally known people

[36] Ephesians 6:12.

whose personalities underwent violent, destructive changes as a result of the study of tantric practices. *Raja* yoga, too, with its miraculous *siddhis*, involves a foray into the occult which is fraught with danger.

But what of *hatha* yoga pure and simple, practised as an end in itself? Here one can speak only from personal experience; and I have to record that I have never come across any case of *hatha* yoga, on its own, producing deleterious effects in a human personality. Many ancient Indian sages looked down on *hatha* yoga because they felt it produced very little in the way of spiritual results; they treated it as a preparatory discipline rather than a means of spirituality in itself. Thus it is possible that in *hatha* yoga we have a neutral set of techniques which have been pressed into the service of Hinduism by their Hindu discoverers, but which can be prised away from that background and used by anyone without ill effect. No-one, after all, refuses to use the photocopier because it was invented by an amateur occultist.

Practically, though, there may be other considerations to bear in mind, and those are dealt with in the appendix. In the meantime, some readers may be becoming impatient. 'All right,' I can imagine them saying, 'you've demonstrated that Christianity and traditional yoga philosophy are poles apart. But yoga *works*. Yogis do have experiences which convince them that they've contacted their true Self, that God has revealed Itself to them. Who's to say that the Christians are right and the yogis are wrong?'

In other words: what is a spiritual experience? What do we mean by 'union with God'?

6
Union with God?

What exactly is a 'spiritual experience'? How do we know when we have had one? The typical answer of mystics down through the centuries has been, 'You will just *know*. Spiritual experiences cannot be reduced to any other terms. You cannot ask for logical proof or chemical analysis; but somehow, in the depths of your being, you will be convinced.'

The only problem with this is that Hitler 'just knew' six million Jews had to die, and the Yorkshire Ripper 'just knew' he had to kill prostitutes. Unexamined intuitions can be dangerous. Any 'spiritual experience' which depends simply on a feeling inside, or a strange physiological event, needs to be looked at more closely; it is possible that there may be alternative explanations of it.

The Divine Light Mission, a Hindu group who enjoyed wide success in the West in the early seventies, believe that contact with the impersonal God within can be made by having the 'divine light experience'. Initiation into the group involves having one's 'third eye' opened (there is a Hindu belief that each of us has a third eye, capable of spiritual perception, situated at the top of the nose) and this happens when the Guru Maharaj Ji or one of his representatives thrusts his fingers into the acolyte's eyes and applies pressure to the optic nerve. A blinding light is (not surprisingly) immediately seen by most people.

The Divine Light 'premies' who have had this experience can be very smug, superior people. They have seen God; you have only theories about him! But then the same experience can be had, with no spiritual trappings whatsoever, by *anyone* who learns the technique of eyeball-pinching. Is this a genuine contact with the divine, or just a normal physical phenomenon?

Hare Krishna devotees sometimes testify that during chanting they find the *mantra* changing its properties. In other words, they begin to hear with their ears a different sound to the one they are making with their lips. But again, there is nothing necessarily spiritual about this:

> In fact psychologists know that when a word or brief phrase is repeated over and over again, it begins to change its characteristics in a peculiar way. This phenomenon... anyone can demonstrate to himself with a tape recorder and an endless loop of tape.... [1]

[1] Christopher Evans, *Cults of Unreason* (London, 1973), p. 243.

It *may* be a spiritual experience; but it *need* not be. Other explanations are possible. Unfortunately it is all too easy to blur the distinction between 'my experience' and 'my interpretation of the experience', and forget that other interpretations might be equally valid. Dr Fritjof Capra, for instance, is an Austrian physicist whose book *The Tao of Physics* has been enormously powerful in urging the view that Eastern, monistic philosophy is 'a consistent and relevant philosophical background to the theories of contemporary science'.[2] But he has arrived at his conclusions, not through reasoned argument, but ultimately because of an experience in which he 'just knew':

> I was sitting by the ocean one late summer afternoon, watching the waves rolling in and feeling the rhythm of my breathing, when I suddenly became aware of my whole environment as being engaged in a gigantic cosmic dance... I 'saw' the atoms of the elements and those of my body participating in this cosmic dance of energy, I felt its rhythm and 'heard' its sound, and at that moment I *knew* that this was the Dance of Shiva, the Lord of Dancers worshipped by the Hindus.[3]

On the face of it, there is no reason why such an experience should not convince Dr Capra of a completely different philosophy of nature -- the Elizabethan concept of the 'Great Chain of Being', say. A sceptic having the same experience might have related it to nothing more than the fact that he had been altering his states of perception chemically with drugs (as, in fact, Capra had). The experience is not self-authenticating; different sorts of interpretation are all possible. Mark Albrecht and Brooks Alexander comment tartly, 'It becomes clear that Dr Capra is not reasoning from premise to conclusion. He is not proposing a theory but announcing a revelation.'[4]

[2] Fritjof Capra, *The Tao of Physics* (London, 1976), p. 25.
[3] *Ibid.*, p. 11.
[4] Mark Albrecht and Brooks Alexander, 'The Sellout of Science', *SCP Journal* August 1978, p. 26.

Turn off your mind
But then, Eastern thinkers would say, the logical mind can never take us to ultimate truth. There comes a point at which it has to be abandoned, and we lose our identity as individuals, merging into the one true reality:

> Turn off your mind relax and float downstream,
> It is not dying, it is not dying,
> Lay down all thought surrender to the void,
> It is shining, it is shining...
>
> Without looking out of my window
> I could know the ways of heaven.[5]

There are several problems with this attitude, however. First, if we abandon logical thought, how do we assess the value of experiences? How can we compare one thing to another? C. E. M. Joad reflected:

> Knowledge is essentially communicable, while feeling is not... It is for precisely this reason that the testimony of mystical experience in religion carries so little weight with non-mystics... knowledge is of something other than and external to itself, whereas feeling reports nothing but the fact of the feeling. Knowledge, in short, involves a reference to something else, namely, that which is known; feeling does not.[6]

Second, is it really a worth-while human aim to seek to lose one's individuality and merge into an impersonal essence? 'A condition in which I shall cease to think,' commented Joad, 'to feel as an individual or, indeed, to *be* an individual, is a condition in which *I* shall cease to be at all. Now why should I hope or seek to realise such a condition, unless I take my individual personality to be of no account?'[7] Whatever our view of reality, we have to live

---

[5] Song by the Beatles; quoted by Colin Chapman, *The Case for Christianity* (Tring, 1981), p. 199.
[6] C. E. M. Joad, *Recovery of Belief* (London, 1952), pp. 97–98.
[7] *Ibid.*, p. 174.

as if our separate, individual personalities mattered; physically, mentally, emotionally, we *are* distinct from other beings, and there is no practical way of living that fails to take this into account. And even if we believe the material world is unreal, *maya,* that will not save us from being run over by a very solid bus should we walk in front of it.

In practical, daily living, logic is not a hindrance but a help. Human beings have made advances in science, technology, philosophy, ethics and art by using their minds; why must they abandon their most useful practical ally as soon as they enter the world of the spirit?

Anyway, if 'all is One', how do we differentiate between true and false, good and evil? If everything is to be accepted as an aspect of the one great whole, where does morality start? And if God is in everything, and everything is a part of God – does the word 'God' actually *mean* anything? Denis Alexander shrewdly observes:

> Another problem with pantheism – the view that God is identical with everything – is that it is difficult to find out what the word really means. The word 'pan' means all. 'Theism' is the belief in a personal, all-powerful, creator God. But when you put the two together they are in fact mutually exclusive. If you believe in a personal God then you cannot at the same time believe that he is the same thing as the whole of impersonal nature. Of course if you have been influenced by a culture with a theistic view of God, then the word pantheism would give an illusion of meaning...But really this is cheating, because there is no real basis...for believing that there is anything personal or special about nature at all.[8]

What we are saying then, is that the experiences provided by Eastern religion – the experiences typical of yoga's 'spiritual' quest – are not necessarily spiritual at all, because there are other possible explanations for them, and logical difficulties involved in accepting the view of reality they suggest. But why do such experiences *seem* to so many people to validate themselves? Why are they so powerful?

[8] Denis Alexander, *Beyond Science* (Berkhamsted, 1972), p. 62.

And what is the attraction of them for so many human beings?

Two possible answers spring to mind. First, there could be a simple psychological basis to mystical experience. Studies in the structure of consciousness show that the two lobes of the brain perform different functions. The left lobe is predominantly concerned with logical, analytical reasoning; the right lobe with intuition and spatial awareness. If the functions of the left lobe can be de-emphasized temporarily, strange changes of consciousness can take place.

Aleister Crowley once forced a film actress, Elizabeth Fox, to spend a month sitting on a cliff-top, eating only bread and drinking only water. 'At first she suffered agonies of boredom; then, towards the end of the month, she sank into a state of ecstatic serenity in which the sea and the sky seemed to become infinitely fascinating. All that had happened is that her over-tense left brain had relaxed its neurotic grip and allowed the right free expression.'[9] Since the left lobe has a great deal to do with our sense of separate identity, it is likely that shutting it off will produce a sense of oneness with all creation, of blending into a cosmic Unity.

Turn outwards

The second possible answer, suggested by Brooks Alexander[10], is that human beings, conscious of their impending death, struggle instinctively to find a pattern within life which will unify and make sense of their fragmented, disparate perceptions. The obvious place to look for such a pattern would be within

> ...some impersonal substrate of 'being' which underlies even the primordial duality of matter and energy, a substrate which is within the cosmos and constitutes its invisible foundation. That such a created substrate does

[9] Colin Wilson and John Grant (eds.), *The Directory of Possibilities* (London, 1981), p. 155.

[10] Brooks Alexander, 'Occult Philosophy and Mystical Experiences', published as a leaflet by Spiritual Counterfeits Project (Berkeley, California, n.d.).

exist seems a reasonable inference from the account of Genesis 1:1–10, in which the Lord reveals that the initial stage of cosmic formation was a state which possessed true created existence, but was 'formless and void', that is, 'without determinate structure'...If it is true that human 'consciousness' is itself an instrument of perception which is capable of making contact with the subtle and unstructured basis of its own created existence (and there seems no Biblical reason for denying it), we can see that this latent...possibility offers a form of unification that is naturally appealing to fallen man.[11]

This seems to fit well with the New Testament's analysis of what has gone wrong with the human search for God. 'They became futile in their thinking and their senseless minds were darkened...they exchanged the truth about God for a lie and worshipped and served the creature rather than the Creator.'[12]

The trouble with Eastern types of mysticism is that they turn us inwards to look for God inside ourselves, leaving man (to quote Déchanet) 'a prisoner of his psyche, of his "self", with neither the prospect nor the hope nor the possibility of soaring up towards Another, towards a living God'.[13] The Bible's solution is markedly different. God exists, but he is not within us; our problem is that the evil and wrongdoing of the human heart keeps him out. He does not want us to blend impersonally into him, but to experience a free, creative friendship with him, in which we retain our individuality, our thinking, critical minds, our personal characteristics.

How does this become possible? Not through a life of spiritual exercises and ascetic struggles. None of us is able to rehabilitate himself sufficiently for the acquaintance of a God of perfection. (Which, incidentally, is a much more realistic perspective on the fallibility of human beings than the wild claims of total sainthood often made for experi-

---

[11] *Ibid.*, pp. 3–4.   [12] Romans 1:21, 25.
[13] J.-M. Déchanet, *Christian Yoga*, p. 14.

enced yogis.) But what man could not do for himself, God did for him:

> For Christ also died for sins once for all, the righteous for the unrighteous, that he might bring us to God.[14]

Because Jesus Christ was willing to die in my place and take upon himself the consequences of my wrongdoing, I can now have a new relationship with God which opens my life up to the transforming power of the Holy Spirit. All I have to do is accept God's forgiveness, and turn my life over to him to direct.

How do I know that this experience is not as imaginary as those we have been criticizing? Because it does not depend on a new, unprecedented mode of consciousness which alters my normal experience of the world, and is open to several different interpretations; but simply fulfils my life – my normal, thinking, conscious life – on so many levels that its presence is undeniable. I begin to find in myself a new desire, which I never had before, to serve God, to love others, to give myself away; I experience a new power to overcome temptations; and, just in case I should begin to feel that these things are purely emotional or psychologically self-produced, I start to notice God at work in my external circumstances too – answering prayer, shaping my daily circumstances, bringing about so many 'coincidences' that all rules of chance are shattered.

The yoga systems of the East command respect. The brilliance of Patanjali and Shankara; the literary skill of the writers of the *Gita* and the *Brihadaranyaka Upanishad*; the sheer self-induced discipline of so many yogis and swamis, Buddhist monks and Sufi mystics – these things are undeniable, and honestly deserve our tribute. They represent some of the greatest efforts of the human spirit.

But they must not be allowed to become a substitute for reality. They must not become a spiritual side-turning which diverts us from the main road of truth.

For the truth can be known.

[14] 1 Peter 3:18.

Appendix:
Reacting to yoga

What should Christians do about yoga classes held in their neighbourhood? Should they campaign against them, ignore them completely, or even join in?

It should be obvious from our earlier description that most of the groups teaching yoga in Britain today are dedicated to teaching the underlying Hindu philosophy, as well as the basic *asanas,* and therefore are involved, consciously or otherwise, in subtly altering the religious world-view of those who submit to their teaching. Even the British Wheel of Yoga, with its strenuous claims of neutrality, incorporates all sorts of elements of Hindu philosophy into its thinking in a chaotic and muddle-headed way ('Yoga teaches that all people are One, that all are One with God and that all religions are true...'[1]).

Further, even if only *hatha* yoga is taught, the connections to other forms of yoga are stressed, and popular magazines such as *Yoga Today* endeavour to awaken interest in more esoteric varieties. *Yoga Today* also carries a large number of articles explicitly teaching Hindu or Buddhist concepts.

It would seem to me quite unacceptable for a Christian to compromise himself by involvement in such a group, and important that he should be able to explain clearly why he disagreed with it. Dark mutterings about demonic influences are not enough. In fact, if *hatha* yoga is a gateway into the demonic (which on the basis of practical experience I doubt), it is not a very obvious or important one, and evidence for the theory is hard to find. We are on much safer ground arguing on the basis of yoga's implicit, underlying philosophy.

How can Christians best help people who are involved in yoga practice but honestly searching for God? First, it has to be appreciated that many dedicated practioners of yoga manifest a self-discipline and self-mastery which puts the lives of many Christians to shame. This needs to be acknowledged. And, it goes without saying, the Christian

[1] British Wheel of Yoga, *Yoga Handbook* (Ilford, n.d.), p. 2.

who will be best equipped to bear witness to yogis will be the one to whom spiritual disciplines, meditation and self-sacrifice are not just words, but form part of their own experience.

If the form of yoga being practised involves submission to a guru, there are more problems. The guru is generally seen only as a catalyst, not someone who gives the truth to the disciple but who helps the disciple to awaken it within his own life; yet nevertheless a guru can have tremendous personal influence over the life and opinions of his followers. It is important to be very sensitive to this.

It is also important to bear in mind the possibility of some kind of occult overhang, if the person concerned is involved in one of the more explicitly mind-transforming or magical forms of yoga. A good Christian book on the subject, such as J. Stafford Wright's *Understanding the Supernatural*, is required reading.

But the most important barriers to Christian communication tend to be two attitudes which the practice of yoga, as normally taught, naturally inculates. The first is the view that all religions are true in a relative way, that truth exists wherever you can find it, that no one path can claim exclusive rights to validity. The second is the idea that experience counts for more than argument. Logic and rationality can advance only so far; conviction comes only by direct experiment. We need to be able to show *why* we believe that Christianity is unique, without sounding arrogant and intolerant; and we need to be able to persuade the yogi to examine his 'experience', asking whether or not it is open to alternative interpretations and is therefore inconclusive. Then, and only then, will we have earned the right to talk about *our* experience.